Food Safety Violation

Violation

The secrets they don't want you to know

By Loura Chong Reid

Table of Contents

Dedication

It is with my deepest gratitude and warmest affection, that I dedicate this book to my wonderful husband who has given me constant support and inspiration in writing this book.

Along with my second mom, who has effortlessly motivated me to do my best.

Preface

Food safety in Jamaica's marketplace is a growing concern like in many other countries around the world. With the increasing movement of foods across the borders, changes in food processing and handling practices and the movement of people across our shores. The possibility of getting a foodborne illness is very high and continues to increase year after year.

According to the World Health Organization, an estimated 600 million people fall ill after eating contaminated food every year with 420,000 succumbing to their illnesses. This is a stunning 1 in every 10 persons around the world.

The effects it has on the country's socio-economic development, health care system, tourism and trade are ginormous. Many skeptics have even reported that the value is unquantifiable, as most times they are unreported, or it is difficult to establish causal relationships between food contamination and resulting illness or death.

In Food Safety Violation: The secrets they don't want you to know, the author reveals the food handling practices of foodservice operators and secrets they don't want the public to know. She points out certain myths and cultural beliefs many people practice, that has contributed significantly to foodborne illness outbreaks in the Jamaican population and also around the world.

As a practicing Environmental Health Officer, she has spent many years, training and developing the knowledge of both food handlers and foodservice operators. This by extension has empowered them to handle food safely and produce only wholesome foods that are fit for human consumption.

She is delighted to publish Food Safety Violation: The secret they don't want you to know, as she recognizes the significance of informing the public of the food handling mal-practices that take place in Jamaica's marketplace. This knowledge will help consumers combat the unscrupulous and deceitful acts that take place in the food industry, and therefore reduce the outbreak of foodborne illnesses and preserve lives.

CHAPTER I

The ugly truth about Jamaica's Marketplace

Introduction

As my four years of study draws closer, I knew all well that my sleepless nights and panic attacks were about to end. The struggles of university life were nothing to play with. I realized then that its either work hard or fail all, but I was relentless, determined and set in my desire to compete and rise to success. It was the passion to learn and my desire to excel in whatever I do, that has morphed me into the Public Health Inspector I am today. Yes, a Public Health Inspector, not a doctor or a lawyer. I, like any other well-established professional, I'm proud and passionate about my job.

As a young professional working in the field of Public Health, I would soon to realize that my job would not limit me to the bounds of my specialty areas; such as water quality, quarantine, vector control, meat hygiene, and food safety, just to name a few.

Rather, I would be challenged in other areas, to develop skills of diverse thinking, good decision making and to master the art of using psychology to complete my assignments.

Quickly acquiring these skills and putting them to work, the results did not take long to follow. I was not just adding value to the lives of others as it relates to Public Health, but also emotional, spiritually and psychologically. As I continue to successfully tackle my assignments day by day, it was starting to become clear to me, the fight to create an impression in the marketplace and impacting the health of the public was never-ending. The more lives I impacted, the more I realized how significant my role is in the profession and to the Jamaican population.

As the Jamaican foodservice industry continues to grow year by year, and with the limited number of Public Health Inspectors in the Island, the challenges to maintain food safety in the marketplace keeps piling up. In spite of this, we are expected to operate with the highest level of integrity in an environment that is greatly influenced by politics, unpredictable uproar of violence and foodservice operators who believe the only duty of the Public Health Inspector is to grant their store a stamp of approval. The Health Department is constantly being blamed for their inefficiency in preventing unscrupulous foodservice operators to dominate the industry, while consumers neglect their responsibility in being wise shoppers.

How could this problem be solved or could it? I pondered night and day. Many have said to me why do you bother yourself with a problem that is way above your pay grade? The answer was distant or maybe I just did not know it, but the only thing I knew then was, if there was a solution I would want to be a part of it.

As the year passes by and I become a more seasoned Public Health Inspector, my perception of the food industry has started to dwindle down a negative path. I was being exposed to the dark side the inner secrets of what takes place behind closed doors. My fear of eating out has grown tremendously, whom could I trust to prepare safe foods for me? No one literally was good enough to meet my requirements of a noble and honest food operator.

It was not very long after I decided to create a website that would provide the public with weekly blogs on pertinent issues like these. I think to myself there are many Jamaicans who are ignorantly shopping in the marketplace because of their lack of information. I believe it's the right of all consumer to be provided with information that will enable them to be more vigilant and conscious of what they are buying to eat. As this platform starting to attract traffic, I realized that people were hungry for knowledge and were willing to act more responsible. Then the idea of this book came to me, all that consumers need to know about the marketplace would now be accessible to them in one package.

As the market for food delivery, take out, online ordering services and fast food services increases in our island, many Jamaicans could be getting more than they pay for. Countless times foods are purchased that are deemed safe, only to be bombarded with excruciating stomach cramps, vomiting, and diarrhea a few hours later. So, who is out there protecting the consumer from that food handler who fails to wash his hand? Or that food services operator who did not prepare the food safely? These are the questions no consumer should ever bother to think about when purchasing foods. There should be a high level of confidence that consumers have when they venture out in the marketplace. One of the ways in which this confidence can be built is by providing them with food safety information that will empower them to be more vigilant and informed customers.

Operators we buy from on a daily

The marketplace is a collective of complex and diverse businesses that supply most of the food consumed by the population. These businesses are from Agricultural, Manufacturing, Food Processing and Preparation, Wholesale and Distribution, Food Servicing and the Grocery sector. As the competition in the food industry becomes fierce by the year, more often than not the priority is being placed on making a profit rather than producing safe foods for consumption. It wasn't until about the year 2011 that I was first faced with realizing this issue.

My very first assignment as a young Public Health Inspector, all the years of information and months of internship was now being put to test. The moment was now, I was to carry out an inspection of a premises that the operator had made application for. On entering the premises, a strong pungent odor welcomes me at the door. I smiled, yes not the typical reaction of an untrained person, but I knew perfectly well it was the scent of spoiled Cod Fish. As eagerly and anxious as I was, to bring to light the display of spoiled food for sale. I remained calm and firmly asked the operator to show me the Codfish she had. The scent was, even more, pronounce as she placed it before me. It was not a pleasant sight, the fish had a pinkish color, moist and showed signs of decay. I, in turn, ask the operator why she had spoiled foods for sale, she replied in a tone of assurance and confidence that the fish only needed to be washed off, as nothing was wrong with it.

This was my first rude awakening of the treacherous and deceitful deeds of foodservice operators in the Jamaica marketplace. This experience amongst many tainted my perception of the food industry, and therefore brings me to the three types of foodservice operators I have encountered in the marketplace. The first is the ignorant operator, just like the example above. This type of operator is clueless about the risk associated with his or her mal-practices when handling food. They have zero knowledge of food safety practices and based their explanation on myths and cultural beliefs.

This type of operator will sieve the weevil from the flour or cornmeal and then put it up for sale. As he or she is ignorant to the fact, that the eggs are able to sieve through the strainer, and in a few days, the food will be infested with weevil once again.

As I work diligently from day to day; my job never seems to disappoint me with the ignorance of most food operator. I remember just a couple years back; a colleague had shared with me a complaint she had received. The operator had encountered some issues with sewer back-up in his facility and the raw sewage from the toilet facility was overflowing in the food storage area. As she investigates with a sense of discreetness, however thoroughly walking through to ascertain the food safety violation that was previously reported, she was astounded to find several bags of rice and sugar on the roof of the building set out to dry. Now, this type of operator is what we call the awfully greedy. They are willing to take extreme measure to ensure they do not lose. Even if it means putting the health of the public at risk. Many times, these types of operators try to butter up to the inspector, by offering free foods or drinks. As a trained professional, I know all too well to avoid any potential conflict is to not accept anything during an inspection.

 The work of the inspector is never done, the quest to ensure that foodservice operators are serving foods that are safe and wholesome, continues at every food premises in the country. We are like society's unsung heroes safeguarding the health of the population, but if you have ever read one of our inspection reports, it could really be some eye-opening stuff. The horror stories of our experiences at times started to sound like the tales your grandmother would tell just before bed. So unbelievable and heart-wrenching that the fear of eating out gripes your minds.

The third and final type of food operators are referred to as the nobles. These operators are always ensuring that their food handling practices are safe. From my experience most times these operators eat from the food they prepare and sell. They are always properly attired even before the inspector shows up and usually washes their hands regularly during the operation. They never think it's safe to handle and prepare foods while sick and keep food safe during storage, preparation, transportation, and distribution. Unlike the awfully greedy operators, the nobles are very aware of the risk associated with food safety violation and makes the conscious decision to only produce safe foods.

In most instances, if not always only one inspection is required to deem their premises safe for selling foods.

Food safety myths and misconceptions consumers believe

Myth" which derived from the Greek word mythos, which means tale or story is one of the things that has created some level of controversy around the topic of food safety in our Island. Like in many other cultures, the Jamaican people have their own perception of food safety. It is believed also that it's our traditional practices when preparing and handling food that has caused us to escape the dreadful hands of foodborne illnesses when compared to other countries.

It is customary in our culture to overcook our foods, wash our raw meats with vinegar or lime and to eat our food when its steaming hot. These food handling practices, even though seems trivial to the ignorant and untrained persons are key practices that reduce the microbial load on what could possibly be a highly contaminated food.

On the contrary, whilst these practices are impactful to us not having such high incidents of foodborne illnesses, there are still a number of beliefs that are engraved in our culture that has caused us to fall ill from consuming unsafe foods.

Ice don't carry germs

One such myth, if not the most commonly echoed amongst Jamaicans, is that "ice don't carry germs." I must admit that I was once among the ignorant in just a few years back, but I have now gained knowledge that has shifted my way of thinking. Additionally, it is funny how illustrating a dramatic scenario of consuming dirty ice can bring about that woo-ha! Moment in someone.

It was about my second health education training, that I discovered the art of illustrating to my audience why ice can and will get you sick if it is unsafe. It's always fun to see the expression on my audience faces when I described the scenario of freezing sewage water and then consider it safe to consume, as it is ice. They are usually astounded and sickened by the mere imagination of my example.

 Freezing contaminated water will not kill most microorganisms, but rather inactivate them. However, when the ideal condition presents itself, e.g. taking the product from the refrigerator and storing it on the countertop, then microorganisms will start to grow and metabolize again.

Therefore, it is not advisable for anyone to be consuming ice, icy drinks or other icy product if he or she deemed any form of contamination. As such practice will for certain get them sick.

The five-second rule

Another well repeated and practice myth that many Jamaicans do is the five-second rule. This is simply picking up food after it has been dropped and thus exposed to contamination, within five seconds. Within this period the food is deemed safe to eat. According to a paper published in the journal of applied biology, five-seconds is way too long. Microorganisms adhere to food almost immediately when dropped. After five-seconds, they found that the food had acquired anywhere between 150-8000 bacteria and if left for a minute the number will be ten times greater

It is believed that the food is safe because most times the surface the food falls on looks clean. Rather, it's important that we note, floors make great homes for bacteria and other disease-causing microorganisms.

Working in the food service industry, the five-second rule is one of the most common mal-practices I encounter on a daily basis. Many food handlers while working in the food area, would willingly ignore the safety of the food that has fallen to the ground. They would quickly pick up the food and continue with their task.

It's never wise to eat food that has fall on a dirty surface, as it could get you ill.

If it looks and smells good, it's safe

This brings me to my next myth that most persons believe. "If it smells good and looks good it's safe to eat." This like the other myths can result in severe health risks or even death when practiced. It's critical that all consumers are aware that we cannot see or smell microorganisms. What we see on foods when they reach a stage of spoilage is the by-product of the microbes' activities. Hence food can be very unsafe but looks perfectly well.

In some cases, it can take a total 10 microbes to get an individual sick. With such a small number of organisms on the food, they will not produce enough by-product such as slime, gas or acids to indicate any changes in the natural form of the food. Therefore, an individual consuming such food that might be contaminated with a very virulent microbe will have no tell-tale sign to know the food is unsafe to consume. In essence, using smell or taste to assess the safety of a food is not recommended and should never be practiced.

Storing hot foods in the refrigerator

Storing hot foods in the refrigerator is a very common practice in the food industry and also amongst consumers. Many are of the impression that a hot pot of food, when stored in the fridge, will be safe, as the food is being stored at a safe temperature.

Putting a hot container in a refrigerator will change its temperature. As a result, the food stored will be exposed to a temperature that will cause microorganisms to multiple in the food.

This will result in the food becoming unsafe and may even show signs of spoilage, such as slimes and a foul odor.

Wearing of gloves

"Workers who wear gloves while handling foods keep my food safe from germs." This is another myth that is strongly believed by consumers, to the point where they would even request for the food handlers to wear gloves while preparing their food. If consumers were to know the staggering truth behind their belief, they would not want to see another glove in the restaurant they eat. It is not that the wearing of gloves is not important.

Glove wearing serves its purpose best when a food handler cuts his or her hands and need to keep their hands from contaminating the food. Wearing the glove by a healthy worker creates a false sense of safety in their minds. Their brains are basically sending a message that their hands are clean, as a result, there is no need to wash their hands as frequently as possible during food handling and preparation. Too many times during my inspection of food handling premises are food handlers observed scratching several parts of their body, touch and handle various foods, without the slightest thought to change their gloves and wash their hands. Gloves can be a useful tool, but they are only helpful if the food handler is conscientious in the first place.

The types of consumers we are

As the marketplace busies with people conducting a hive of activities, many are clueless to the dangers that linger in the very same place they go to purchase foods that are safe and wholesome. It's interesting to see, as Jamaicans how we choose our foods. I figured it may not be different from other cultures however, it's a very important topic that needs to be brought to the fore. Consumers are always casting the blame for the increase in foodborne illnesses on food services operators, but the fact of the matter is they are equally contributing to the food safety problem facing Jamaica.

According to an article on the University of Minnesota website, titled, Prepared Food for Health and Safety. Written by Barb Leonard in 2016. Foodborne illnesses don't just come from restaurants. In fact, they usually come from bad food preparation, serving, and storage at home.

The very same consumers who complain about the ineffectiveness of the health department with the closure of certain premises are the very same consumers who would go to purchase foods from these premises. I remember most recently while conducting one of our weekly food handlers' training, a trainee had to strike up a very controversial discussion regarding the food handling practices of a particular ethnic group. While I listen to the discriminatory and bashing comments made towards these people, I had an epiphany. If as consumers, we experience such horrific food handling dismays when purchasing foods from these operators, why do we continue to buy from them? There it was, the perfect time to interject and to get the answer to my question.

Without a tip of hesitation, my answer was thrown right back at me. Cheap! yes that's was the reply, as sad as it sounds, it was the truth.

This, therefore, brings me to the three types of consumers I come in contact with on a daily basis. The first is the cheap consumer, these types of buyers give no thought about where they buy food or the safety of it. It's like the proverb most Jamaicans jokingly throw around, "wah nuh kill fatten!" naive to the danger of consuming unsafe food. My first experience with this ignorant belief, was a couple years back when I was called to conduct a foodborne illness investigation. A person had bought a box of rice and peas and chicken from a vendor who apparently wasn't practicing safe food handling. This act even though seems innocent resulted in the consumer paying the cost with his life. Never have I ever thought, that someone could just so easily lose his or her life over eating a mere box of food. This was the reality, the ugly truth of the foodservice industry. It's not that being cost-effective is a bad thing, but it's rather stupid to just base the safety of our food on the price they are sold for.

The second type of consumer is called the convenience buyer, how many of you can relate to this type? The convenient buyer will purchase foods from places that will not take them out of their way. For example, in locations that are closest to their place of residence or work. The problem with this concept is that the safety of the food is not their priority, but rather where would create an ease for them or where they could be in and out in a minute. In many instances, these types of consumers will be the ones who would buy food from an unsanitary food place then go and make a complaint about what they saw. The thing that they are most times naïve to, is that buying food from an unsanitary place could put them at risk of getting a foodborne illness or even worst death.

A perfect experience I had, was a complaint my colleagues and I had received of a food service operator selling expired foodstuffs. On our arrival at the premises, a number of consumers were purchasing items. After a thorough inspection of the premises, the complaint was validated as several boxes of foods were condemned and the establishment was closed for other food safety violations. With the sign of closure being erected, consumers were very distraught as they did not want to go elsewhere to make their purchases. This location was convenient for them despite how unsanitary and unsafe the environment and foods were.

So, you see many Jamaicans are not thinking that the safety of the foods they eat contribute significantly to their health. While purchasing foods I usually think of this proverb, "you are what you eat!" As a result, consuming safe foods will preserve your health.

To even reiterate the carelessness of some consumers when they purchase foods, a group of Public Health Inspectors and myself was inspecting a certain establishment that was reported to have an unpleasant odor emitted from a section of the store. As the inspection was being conducted, I overheard a few consumers saying to one of my colleagues, "Uno lock ye dung! dem too nasty." However, they continue to proceed to the counter to cash their items.

Puzzling! Oh, but it's the truth, I had to address them and asked why would they still buy from a place that did not meet Public Health standard? Long gone are the days when consumers would stop purchasing when the inspector walks in to conduct an inspection. Or would only buy foods from food service establishments that the inspector renders safe to purchase from. As consumers, we need to be more vigilant and proactive in the marketplace. If we do not purchase from these unsanitary premises they will be forced to adhere to Food handling regulation and only sell safe and fit foods.

The final type of consumer is the conscientious buyer or the safe buyers. These types of consumers will put safety at the top of their list. It's not to be mistaken that these consumers are not shopping with an economical mindset and convenience, however, at the end of the day, they will only purchase from sanitary food premises. This is the type of consumer I desire all Jamaicans to be.

For the few persons who might be asking this question, "but what is a sanitary food store?" A sanitary food store is an establishment that has been inspected and pass by the health department. This establishment is considered safe to sell foods, as it has passed all the critical areas of the food handling regulation.

As consumers, whenever you are purchasing food, you need to be your own inspector. The first thing that you can note in food premises is the environment of the establishment, that is how clean, odorless and well organized the premises is. Secondly, the attire of the staff and their practices. Are they wearing their hair nets and other protective clothing? Are they washing their hands after completing a task or when necessary?

Additionally, you can check for their health certificate, which should be conspicuously placed in the establishment. The health certificate is a pink certificate which is issued by the health department. It is signifying that the premises was inspected and render safe to sell food. Like any other certifying document, the health certificate has an expiry date so, it's also important to look out for that as well.

The conscientious buyers even though seem to be a very small percentage of our population, they are everywhere. This has been proven to me in a not so recent experienced I had at an abattoir or what most Jamaicans would call a butcher shop. As I pull up to the location, a line of customers was eagerly waiting on the outside. Not one to make a purchase before the stamp of approval of the Public Health Inspector. This was amongst many other experienced that I have had where consumer made a conscious decision to buy their foods from a safe source.

 Consumers have a very crucial role to play in an effective food safety system. Remember, the food industry revolves around the purchasing power and decisions of consumers. Therefore, if that power is given to foodservice operators then we will forever lose the battle of foodborne illness outbreak in our Island. it's my hope for all consumers to be more conscious of where they purchase their foods and how safe the foods are.

CHAPTER II

The unspoken Secret

How could it be staler yet more expensive

The food service industry is a well-known lucrative business in Jamaica and around the world. It has been said by many, that to be sure of success, the food industry could be considered one of the ways to quickly get you there. Foods are consumables and are needed to provide nutrients, energy and to sustain life, but if not safely handled could be like a double-edged sword that will shorten the days of the one who dears it.

As we dive into the various food secrets that have been documented in the foodservice industry. The question lingers could we be paying more for foods that are old and stale? The answer is yes! And if as consumers we are not vigilant when purchasing our foods, the implications could be catastrophic.

A very close friend of mine once told me of an experience she had while working for a grocery store operator. She said she was being forced to sell food to the public that was old and infested. In spite of her many attempts to warn consumers, they would still make their purchase, and some would even report her to her manager. The moral of the story is there are many foodservice operators who are involved in the practice of selling food that is stale to the public and have no regrets doing it. Likewise, there are many food handlers who are coerced into these mal-practices because of fear of losing their job.

 In our island, there are many standards and policies which governs the food safety operation in this industry, but quite often the consumer gets a raw deal. As Public Health Inspectors around the country continues to ensure that foodservice operators are serving foods that are safe and wholesome. We crave the keen eyes of the consumers to be more efficient and effective at our job. In the food service industry there are many tricks to the trade. Most food service owner is not in the business because of their passion for food safety, but rather to make a profit. Walking down the aisles of your favorite grocery store, the foods may look good but what happens behind closed door will gross you out.

Despite my many years of experience, it always seems to surprise me the extreme measures food operators are willing to take to make a profit. This was proven to me when I stumbled across a series of video produced by the Canadian Broadcasting Cooperation News, called Marketplace. This series of videos shed light on how grocery store operators tamper with stale and spoil foods to give them a second life. Yes, I know! Deception at its worse and totally unethical.

A supermarket insider reveals how his supervisor would stock up all the brown stale meats from off the shelve, dip them in a little blood to increase its red appearance. These products would then be re-package for sale. In addition, if the meat was close to spoiling, they would either marinate it with spices or sauce to disguise its odor and staleness. In other instances, they would grind old meat with fresh meat to make it appears fresher. As misleading as it sounds the risks are even more heart-wrenching.

The interesting thing about this practice is that in most cases grounded and marinated meats are sold at an increased price when compare to steak cut and fresher meats. This concept is referred to as value-added, so because something is added to the natural product it increases the price. This insider has me thinking, could these unscrupulous and deceptive acts be taking place in Jamaica's Marketplace? As consumers, we are often naïve, and we trust that the foods with put in our supermarket trolley are safe and wholesome for us. No! not in all cases, this is the reason I am going to reiterate my advice, that we need to be our own inspectors when purchasing our food.

The grinding of old meat with fresh meat is never acceptable as old meat that has been mixed with new meat could be loaded with harmful bacteria and their toxins. Another thing to note is that meat in its whole state or steak form could be considered safer when compared to the grounded meat. This is simply because a steak cut would most times have microorganisms on its outer surface whereas for the grounded meat would have the microbes spread throughout the entire product.

There are three sensory properties by which consumers judge the quality of their meat;

appearance, texture, and flavor. The most important property at the time of purchase is the appearance of the product because texture and flavor cannot be evaluated when the product is packaged. Surface discoloration is inevitable and is used as an indicator of freshness. Hence doctoring its appearance after the meat has gone stale will deceive the consumer, and if safe food handling practices and correct cooking temperatures are not adhered to, the results could be very unfavorable.

The risks are even more life-threatening when tamping with foods that are considered high-risk food. If I could give a simple definition of what high-risk foods are, I would say foods that are rich in protein, low in acidic content and high in moisture. So, for e.g. our meats, meat products, dairy, dairy Products, gravy, certain salads, soft cheese just to name a few. To even make it a bit easier for the concept to be clear, I could say any food that can be spoiled easily if left out on the counter or at the danger zone temperature.

To drive home the concept to food handlers, I normally like to ask this question. If I should place a chicken leg and a slice of bread out in the sun or in the danger zone, which one would spoil first? One hundred percent of the time I will get the correct answer.

As it relates to the danger zone, it's a term used in food safety to describe a range of temperatures that bacteria and other microorganisms multiply rapidly. The range of numbers may vary slightly based on the jurisdiction or policy you are reading. However, as it relates to the Public Health Food Handling Regulation 2000 the range is between 4.4 degree Celsius and 63.7 degree Celsius.

Another crucial thing that I believe a lot of consumers are not aware of, is that most foods are contaminated with microorganisms before they even think to purchase them. Contamination could be from the soil, air, poor food handling practices, temperature abuse or even the food natural flora. Therefore, with operators tampering with the foods we purchase from them, is only adding fuel to the fire. They are only making the food become more unsafe for the consumer. I strongly believe in the slogan, your health is your responsibility, but it is very difficult to be responsible when there is deception all around in the marketplace.

Food for thought while picking it from the shelf

Did you know that two-thirds of what you buy in the supermarket you had no intention of buying? This was outlined by consumer expert Paco Underhill, author of Why We Buy: The Science of Shopping. Every aspect of the store layout is so arranged to peak your desires to want to buy from each aisle. To even aid this process stimulating music is being played in each aisle to invoke purchasers to full up their trolley with all that they do not need.

Similarly, to this concept, most supermarkets, and other food store arrange food items to encourage consumers to choose less fresh foods from the shelve. This is because older goods are stock to the front and the fresher ones are at the back. This method is called FIFO which is a stock inventory method or a method in which stock is rotated based on the date in which they were purchased. Most food handlers know this method as the first in first out method.

 This, therefore, means that the usual shelf layout in your favorite food stores is packed to encourage you to always purchase foods with a shorter shelf life. This is so, as most shoppers will just pick from the front of the shelf for the less fresh foods. This concept even though seems unethical is actually a well-encouraged phenomenon in the food industry and the food safety policies and regulations. Packing older foods to the front of the shelf or where shoppers have easy access to them is done to get out the older goods before they become spoiled.

One supermarket insider also revealed that they were instructed to pack fresher foods at the extreme bottom or top, this is because most consumers will not go out of their way to pick foods from these locations. This practice notwithstanding it advantages may be flawed to a certain extent. Reason being, foods that are purchased a week later are not necessarily fresher than foods that were purchased a week ago. There are certain foods like canned food that carries a long shelf life and will be able to remain in food storage longer when compared to dairy products and other high-risk foods. As a result, if the purchasing time is the only factor that is used as an inventory method to place items on shelves then it is highly possible for stale foods that have passed their best before date to be put out for sale.

In other cases where this concept has proven its ineffectiveness, are when two for one promotion is displayed in food stores. Unlike the FEFO inventory method, the FIFO method does not pay much attention to the expiry date, best before dates of food and frequency of sale. Hence, goods are often times not effectively rotated to get out the older goods on time. This inefficiency resulting in food service operators having to take drastic measure to increase sales and quickly get them in the customers' hands.

This reminds me of an encounter I had during one of my food premises inspections. While going through each shelve checking best before dates and the physical condition of the food items on display. I kept finding stale foods that have passed their best before date, in a voice of curiosity and concern, I asked the operator why he had so many stale foods on the shelve? He was stunned, in disbelief, he sorts through item by item to realize the scam he was sold instead of a deal. "That two for one promotion was a scam he screamed!" As his face filled with anger and his eyes slowly transition in a gaze of disappointment.

 He had seen the promotion and thought it was a great deal and therefore purchase an excess of these food items. The frequency of sale in that community was not as rapid, as a result, the short shelf life of the goods would now catch up on him and even worst he would innocently sell them to the public.

It is for this reason why a few food operators are adapting to the FEFO stock management system. What this method means is first expired first out, and basically all foods with an older best before dates are sold first regardless of the date of entry or acquisition. This method if managed effectively with the use of inventory and distribution software could increase the lead time to put out goods so consumers can purchase fresher foods with a longer shelf life.

 it's very crucial that consumers make informed choices when they are purchasing foods. Inspect your foods carefully and check your label and dates. Choose your food items from the extreme back, bottom or top of shelves. Remember there are operators who are not well informed in the management and safety of foods, therefore you have to take the necessary step to preserve your own health.

Best before after its best before

As we venture out in the marketplace week by week, very seldom are consumers taking note of the varying types of dates on foods labels and understanding what each type means. The two most common types of food date that consumers will come across in the grocery stores are the best before date and the use by date.

In our Island Jamaica, the regulatory body that is responsible for checking and assessing dates on food labels is the Bureau of Standard Jamaica.

According to their standard specification for labeling of the food item, each date marks are important and should be presented in a day, month and year format for foods that are to be consumed in three months. For foods that should be consumed three months and beyond the date marked must be presented in the format of month and year, in which each is clearly differentiated.

Well to the untrained consumer it may appear that both dates are inter-changeable used when labeling foods. On the contrary, they are completely different in meaning. A used by date could be considered the most important of the two as it relates to the safety of the food. If you should purchase a food with this date mark, it is simply saying the food is safe to be eaten up to that date, but not after. You will see this type of data on high-risk foods such as milk, dairy product, meats, meat products, salads, baby formulas and some ready to eat items.

In order for the use-by date to be a valid guide, care must be taken to follow storage instructions outlined on the label. For example, refrigerated after opening or keep refrigerated at seven

Degrees Celsius. Therefore, if storage and packaging instructions are not followed, the safety of the food could be compromised before the date.

On the other hand, best before dates are never about the safety of the food but rather its quality. In essence, foods that have passed their best before date, might not be as flavorful and nutritional as when they were fresh but is considered safe to eat. Some food items that are labelled with this date are frozen foods, canned foods, and dried foods.

Despite this clear difference in the best before date and use by date, there have been products such as seafood, deli meats, and soft cheese that are being mislabeled. With these products being placed on shelves with a best before food dates consumers might be misguided in consuming them pass their dates. The reasons these foods should never be consumed after the date marked on the label is because certain pathogens can grow on them and they might taste and smell fine but could be very dangerous.

It could be because of this practice, why persons are insinuated that manufacturers and food operators are doctoring the dates on food labels to give them a new life. This practice even though has not been documented in our country, is a well know food safety concern in other countries. According to an article in the Britain newspaper, The Telegraph, with the headline: How manufacturers secretly change the best before the date on foods. Written by the chief reporter, Andrew Alderson. He stated that Truman Advance Group, of Watnall Road, Hucknall and two of his directors pleaded guilty at Nottingham magistrate court to infringing trade description and food labeling regulations.

He further went on to state that changing labels to be able to keep selling out-of-date products have become big business in Britain, as they struggle to cope with an estimated of 3 billion euro of surplus food every year.

Graham Fisher, the managing director of Food Development United Kingdom, a Hampshire-based food wholesale also outlined in the article that his company often carried out re-labeling work. Despite Mr. Fisher, may get his foods re-analyzed before he carries out his re-labeling process to ensure they are given a bill of health. What about those operators who fail to follow this path? The thought that this process is even being carried out on highly perishable foods and without the knowledge of the consumer is grossly unethical.

Julia Lennard, a senior food researcher with the consumer group in Britain has highlighted that this situation is often times confusing and misleading for the consumer. One example she stated was when food processing plants re-dated unsold raw chicken to retailers up to 20days between slaughter and use-by date without their knowledge.

With retailers buying goods that are already behind their best before and use-by date, and them also tampering with these dates if goods are not sold out in time. This only leaves the consumers getting foods with limited shelf life or even worse spoil goods.

As was noted on the Canadian Broadcasting Cooperation website, there have been several supermarket staff that has reported that they were given instruction by their manager to change the dates on several foods such as, whole cakes that have passed their best before date. These items were then re-packaged in smaller serving size with a new best before date on each serving. In addition, fruit tart is another popular food that has been reported to be re-surfaced with fresh topping and fruits after they have gotten old and moldy. This practice can be very dangerous, as Aspergillus, a very dangerous mold could be growing on the tart, which would not be visible to the naked eyes. Aspergillus microbes produce a micro toxin which can be very fatal over time to consumers

With all these research and investigations being conducted in other countries, it has me thinking could these very same practices be happening under our nose? The interesting thing is, Jamaica does not have a known system in place where reports like these are documented and are made available to the public. A lack of communication and feedback of food safety risks will not only reduce consumers' confidence in the marketplace but also open them to more hazards when shopping.

CHAPTER III

Wisdom in the Marketplace

The art of a wise shopper

With the increased talk about the effects that date marking has on food waste around the world, many manufacturers and regulatory agencies are working together to see how they can tackle this economic and environmental monster. Having so much food goes to waste per year, they believe addressing this issue could also bridge the gap of the millions of people around the world that struggle to find enough food to eat.

A recent study carried out by the European Commission, published in February 2018, estimated that up to 10% of the 88 million tons of food waste generated annually in the EU are linked to date marking on foods. Similarly, according to the New York Times, 60 million metric tons of food is wasted every year in the United States alone. This is worth about $162 billion of food. Thirty-two million metric tons end up in landfills which cost local governments $1.52 billion.

Notwithstanding that this tremendous initiative will contribute significantly to the economy and environmental issues we face, but it is still crucial that the consumer's safety is not being put at risk. As consumers, we need to pay more attention to the labeling and date marking on foods. Make it a priority to understand the meaning of the best before date and use-by date. Ask key question like, are you certified by the health department?

It is imperative to keep in mind the principle most food operators practiced when packing the shelves in the supermarket. FIFO stock rotation, therefore always choose the fresher foods from the back or the extreme bottom. Remember these locations are normally not easily accessible to you, therefore that's where most likely the fresher goods will be placed.

Most food store layout is arranged in such a way for consumers to pick up produce, meat and dairy products before shopping the main aisles, but it is safer to pick up those items last. This is because these high-risk foods should not be off refrigerated temperature for more than two hours or no more than one hour in a very hot environment.

Refrain from buying foods from the cheapest and most convenient source, without ensuring that the premises are safe and food handlers are practicing good food handling habits. Never walk away from the cashier without checking the dates on your foods, especially for your soft cheese, deli meat, poultry, dairy, baby formulas and meats. Most times, they are the foods that will send you in the hospital if you consume them after the date marking on them has expired.

As for two-for-one promotions or promotions where goods are married with others, never purchase these items in excess before checking date. For example, three days or less. It is also a common practice for food items on promotion to be packaged to hide the expiration dates, don't be afraid to ask for assistance in such case to remove packing material to check the dates.

When purchasing freshly prepared foods from food service establishments, such as restaurants pay keen attention to the temperature of the food you receive. The simple concept of keeping hot foods hot and cold foods cold has never proven to be faulty. Holding foods at their correct temperature will reduce the possibility of you getting a foodborne illness.

It has been noted during my years of practice that the two common foods you will likely see stored at the incorrect temperature in most food stores are eggs and cheese. In most instances, they will be seen displayed on shelves rather than in a refrigerated area. Eggs are to be stored at seven-degree Celsius to maintain it prescribed shelf life. When picking your eggs, be sure to check the carton for crack eggs and off odors.

Also pay attention to canned products when picking them from the shelves. Observe for any signs of dents, swollen, leaks or damaged and imperfect labels. According to the FDA, these signs in canned products could indicate Clostridium botulinum contamination that may lead to deadly implications. Labeling must always be written in a language spoken and should be clear in its description. Never purchase foods that are not labelled for you clearly to understand.

When purchasing frozen meats, pay close attention to the color of the ice. Reason being is, meats that have been thawed and re-frozen contain ice that have a red or bloody appearance. This is very crucial because if meat was improperly thawed, there could be a high level of microbes on it which could get you sick.

The secret to be a wise shopper does not only revolve around using your sense of sight. You must be vigilant which involves using as much of your senses as possible. Remember whenever you are in doubt never buy.

The simple guide to safeguarding the health of your consumers

We all know the one thing that drives a business is a profit, but very seldom does food operators focus on the consumers who make the business successful. This vital part of the puzzle is most times tossed to the side while its by-product is pushed to the front. Most foodservice operators continue to fail in their endeavor to retain high credibility and desire from the very ones who aided in the business success. Yes! The most important thing about the marketplace, the thing that stands out and influences the direction of growth or failure in the food industry is the consumers' experience.

When a consumer feels their safety is at risk from the food they buy, mainly because of the low quality and unwholesomeness they will lose the desire to want to buy from that food service operator. Without saying, we can predict what the outcome will look like. As a result, in order for foodservice operators to continually strive and excel in the marketplace, they would want to keep this small token of wisdom in mind.

To control foods' safety and quality, there are several different processes food operators must keep in mind. With proper care and proactiveness practiced in all these areas, there is a high chance they will be selling safe and quality foods to the public. The following processes are; purchasing of goods, packaging, storage, preparation and proper training of staff.

The very first question a food service operator should ask before they make their purchase is, am I purchasing from an approved source? If in doubt never take the chance. An approved source is always certified by all the regulatory agencies and is always willing to prove their legitimacy.

Ensure that all foods are stamped and properly labelled by the respective agencies. Example, Bureau of Standard Jamaica and the Public Health Department. As the food service operator, develop a relationship with your supplier, get to know their food safety practice. This could include reviewing their most recent inspection report.

When receiving foods, it's very important that the labels are attached and can be clearly read, there should be no signs of pest infestation and the packaging should be clean and in good conditions. There should be no abnormal color or odor observed. If products require refrigeration during transportation, the temperature at which the food is received should be in accordance with the prescribed holding temperature.

Observe the condition of the vehicle in which the food is being transported. The vehicle should be clean and odorless. The package and layout of food in the vehicle and how the worker handles the foods is also very important. It's a regular practice for workers to sit on the foods, put their dirty clothes and shoes on them and handle them in an unsafe manner.

Another important thing that most foodservice operators take for granted is the time they receive goods. Receival of goods should be scheduled to facilitate an easy flow of storing of high-risk foods immediately, and packing of other goods in their respective locations as soon as possible. Therefore, ensure adequate staff is available at the time of receival.

The lack of this practice is commonly observed during my inspection of food stores. Operators are normally observed selling from their freshly received goods, as they are usually easily accessible to them. This practice most time results in older goods not being sold as quickly and sometimes expired in the store. Most critically are the foods that are to be stored immediately after being received such as the high-risk foods which are of great concern. A break in the cold chain or hot chain could result in serious health implication for the consumer. This is because exposing these types of foods to the danger zone temperatures will result in rapid growth of bacteria and other microorganisms in the food, which could get them sick.

Another critical step that operators should pay attention to is the storage of goods. Not all foods are stored in the same storage area. Reason being different foods require different storage condition to maintain their shelf life. Goods are normally divided into three storages; cold, dry and frozen. Dry storage area normally has foods that have a longer shelf life and can be stored at room temperature. This area must be free from pest and mold growth. Well ventilated to prevent moisture or sweating of the area and the foods. All food items must have a layout where there is walking space between each row, they should be off the ground and ceiling and away from walls. Remember only foods should be stored in this area, no clothing, old furniture, and equipment. It is a food storage area not a changing room, garage or a locker.

It has also been noted that operators, would place rat poisons and baits in these areas, this is a no! no! Rats are known to take their foods and hide, having poison in the food storage area, will result in them contaminating the food with these chemicals. As a result, stick traps and other devices that will hold them stationary are the only recommendations.

Cold storage is mainly for foods that are to be kept at a refrigerated temperature, for example, your produce, eggs, cheese, and milk. The most basic rule when storing foods in this area is that cooked or ready-to-eat products must be stored at the top while raw products stored at the bottom. This reasoning is that the prepared food would have already gone through a cooking process which would reduce any form of contaminants, as a result rendering the food safer than the uncooked food. Always store foods in their designated area of the refrigerator, as certain products like dairy items take on the odor of their environment or foods they are stored with.

For frozen foods like your meats and poultry should be stored at −18°C (0°F) or lower. If this temperature is not maintained, then food can become discolored and lose nutrient content. Finally, create a temperature schedule to monitor the temperature of this area, to maintain the safety of these foods.

When preparing food, the aim is to keep the food safe until it is served to the consumer. Therefore, every action taken in the preparation processes must be done to minimize contamination of the food. Taking the relevant precautionary measures such as, washing hands frequently, cook foods to correct temperature, don't mix hot and cold foods together, wear protective clothing while handling the food, will prevent foodborne illness.

Food handlers can carry germs on their skin, in their hair, on their hands, and in their digestive systems or respiratory tracts. Unless workers are proactive and understand the basic food protection principles, they may unintentionally contaminate fresh produce and fresh-cut produce, food contact surfaces, water supplies, or other workers, and thereby, create the opportunity to transmit foodborne illness.

Basic food protection practices related to worker health and hygiene fall into two categories, disease control, and cleanliness. (FDA,2018)

Therefore without proper training and monitoring of staff in these areas, the risk of getting the consumer sick is exponentially high.

Deficiencies in the food safety system

Although food safety is the responsibility of everyone, from producers to consumers, Health and other the regulatory agencies have an essential role to play in safeguarding the health of the population. As the era of new interventions and technology welcomes itself in the 21st century, new challenges to food safety will continue to emerge. These problems will become more pronounce largely because of; changes in our food production and supply, including more imported foods, changes in the environment leading to food contamination, better detection, new and emerging bacteria, toxins, and antibiotic resistance, changes in consumer preferences and habits and changes in the tests that diagnose foodborne illness. (CDC, 2017).

With the myriad of challenges that come with coordinating an effective food safety programme, Jamaica continues to lag behind as it relates to appointing a single agency or ministry to coordinate their food safety programme. According to the National food safety policy,

2003 this responsibility is mainly shared amongst Agriculture and Fisheries, Health, and Industry Investment & Commerce and their respective department/divisions or agencies. Having several ministries or agency sharing this responsibility has resulted in the overlapping of responsibility, variations in the interpretations and enforcement of laws. This is because each agency involved is operating under their set of legislation.

According to an article published by the Jamaica Information Service, the Permanent Secretary in the Ministry of Agriculture and Fisheries, Donovan Stanberry, pointed out that the establishment of the Food Safety Agency is expected to significantly reduce, if not eliminate, challenges such as duplication and simplifying the processes involved in importing foods and monitoring the quality of same.

"When you have one agency, you are better able to use your resources. Everything will be consolidated in one place." With all the supporting data that proves the importance of having one agency coordinating the food safety programme, yet the country continues to waste resources and time on having this programme shared amongst the ministries.

Food safety is a crucial aspect of a country's Public Health programme. Having consumers getting ill from purchasing unsafe foods will contribute significantly to the cost of the health care system, economic development, and the country's image. While there were no estimates of the total costs of these diseases at the regional level, the available data indicated that $700,000 to $19 million in annual health costs is spent in the Caribbean. It has been estimated to cost the United States around $7 billion per year for food safety incident.

In recognition of the deficiencies in sharing the food safety programme, there is also a lack of information that is made accessible to consumers as it relates to the violation committed by foodservice operators. With the present food safety programme, consumers are only provided with the sanitary inspection status of the food premises and not the violations committed during their recent inspection. Food establishments can be issued a stamp of approval without meeting all the requirements outlined in the food inspection report. These violations are usually non-critical however should be accessible to the public.

An inspection grading system could combat this issue, as it will allow consumers to have a greater insight into the practices and violation of a food store or restaurant.

This system is practiced by other countries around the world and can provide a framework for our Island food safety coordinators to adopt and improved on. An example of how this system works is by allotting a score to a restaurant or food store based on the number of violations. A Restaurant with a score between 0 and 13 points earn an A grade, those with 14 to 27 points receive a B and those with 28 or more earns a C. This grade is allotted at the end of the inspection, after the inspector totals the points. The lower the score, the better.

Providing this information on a website that is accessible to the public, along with having food service operators display their grade at the front of their establishment can increase the consumer's confidence. Consumer's confidence is a very vital commodity in the food industry and should never be taken for granted. According to the report, "Building Trust in What We Eat," by Sullivan Higdon & Sink Food Think, only 17 percent of consumers trust food companies. It continues to outline that, much of this mistrust stems from little knowledge about how food is produced, as well as consumer perceptions that food makers lack transparency and place profits above values.

Failing to please the consumer can have dire implication on the food industry and more so the economy. Hence it is crucial that the authorities involved in appointing a single agency to coordinate the country's food safety programme hasten their steps. In addition, creating a programme where more pertinent information is accessible to consumers and food operators making a conscious decision to sell safe food, is very critical to having an efficient system. These suggestions should have a positive effect on the food industry and its relationship with consumers.

In conclusion, I hope this information was of some help, and there will be a tremendous reduction in foodborne illness outbreaks in our Island.

References

The author would like to thank the following organizations and websites for contributing to the information that was used in the writing of this book.

1.   National Food Safety Policy, 2003
http://www.moa.gov.jm/AboutUs/departments/National_Food_Safety_Policy.pdf

2.   Malik Altaf Hussain and Christopher O. Dawson, 2013 Economic Impact of Food Safety Outbreaks on Food Businesses
https://www.ncbi.nlm.nih.gov/pmc/articles/PMC5302274/

3.   World Health Organization, 2015 Unsafe foods cause over 200 illnesses
http://www.jamaicaobserver.com/news/Unsafe-foods-cause-over-200-illnesses--says-WHO_18708098

4.   New York City Health (n.d), How We Score and Grade

https://www1.nyc.gov/assets/doh/downloads/pdf/rii/how-we-score-grade.pdf

5. European Commission. (n.d). Date marking and food waste

https://ec.europa.eu/food/safety/food_waste/eu_actions/date_marking_en

6. Ron Nixon, 2015 Food Waste Is Becoming Serious Economic and Environmental Issue, Report Says https://www.nytimes.com/2015/02/26/us/food-waste-is-becoming-serious-economic-and-environmental-issue-report-says.html

7. Canadian Broadcasting Cooperation New. 2015. Best before dates: How supermarkets tamper with your food (CBC Marketplace)

https://www.youtube.com/watch?v=ZxCT_D6HBd8&t=1108s

8. R. Dhananjayan I. Y. Han J. C. Acton P. L. Dawson. 2006. Growth Depth Effects of Bacteria in Ground Turkey Meat Patties Subjected to High Carbon Dioxide or High Oxygen

Atmospheres.
https://academic.oup.com/ps/article/85/10/1821/1534207

9.   Jamaica Information Service. 2010.Government to Establish Food Safety Agency

https://jis.gov.jm/government-to-establish-food-safety-agency/

10.   Centers for Disease Control and Prevention. 2017. Challenges in Food Safety.
https://www.cdc.gov/foodsafety/challenges/index.html

11.   Lindsey Jahn. 2014. Putting Trust on the Table: Boosting Consumer Confidence in the Food Industry
https://www.manufacturing.net/blog/2014/02/putting-trust-table-boosting-consumer-confidence-food-industry

12.   World Health Organization. 2017. Food Safety.

http://www.who.int/news-room/fact-sheets/detail/food-safety

13.   U.S Food and Drugs Administrator. 2018. Guidance for Industry: Guide to Minimize Microbial Food Safety of Fresh-cut Fruits and Vegetables

https://www.fda.gov/Food/GuidanceRegulation/GuidanceDocumentsRegulatoryInformation/ProducePlantProducts/ucm064458.htm

About the Author

Loura Chong Reid is a Public Health Inspector for the Ministry of Health in the island of Jamaica.

She also is the co-owner of Jamaica Health Tips Online which is the number one Health Tips website for the island of Jamaica.

Loura is married with one son and does voluntary work in her community sharing her knowledge of environmental health with others.